THE MIGRAINE DIET GUIDE

A Complete Diet Guide for People with Migraine Attacks

MONIKA SHAH

ALSO INCLUDES

(MIGRAINE SAFE & UN-SAFE FOODS, GROCERY SHOPPING LIST
AND EATING OUT TIPS & GUIDELINES)

Production Credits
Cover design by Aaskformore
Text design by Monika Shah
Edited by Monika Shah
Printed by CreateSpace, On-Demand Publishing, LLC

Disclaimer
The information contained in this book is not designed to replace or take the place of any form of medicine or professional medical advice. The information in this book has been provided for educational and entertainment purposes only.

The information contained in this book has been compiled from sources deemed reliable, and it is accurate to the best of the Author's knowledge; however, the Author cannot guarantee its accuracy and validity and cannot be held liable for any errors or omissions. Changes are periodically made to this book. You must consult your doctor or get professional medical advice before using any of the suggested remedies, techniques, or information in this book.

Upon using the information contained in this book, you agree to hold harmless the Author from and against any damages, costs, and expenses, including any legal fees potentially resulting from the application of any of the information provided by this guide. This disclaimer applies to any damages or injury caused by the use and application, whether directly or indirectly, of any advice or information presented, whether for breach of contract, tort, negligence, personal injury, criminal intent, or under any other cause of action.

You agree to accept all risks of using the information presented inside this book. You need to consult a professional medical practitioner in order to ensure you are both able and healthy enough to participate in this program.

To all those who are suffering from
Migraine Attacks

CONTENTS

A Message for Readers!

Live Migraine Free by eating right and following a healthy Lifestyle

This book has been specifically designed and written for people who suffer from Migraine attacks time to time and seriously looking for easy to follow methods to keep this unbearable disease away. Apart from taking medications prescribed by the doctor, it is extremely important to eat the right type of foods, as some foods may trigger Migraine attacks. This book will not only help you in identifying foods that may trigger Migraine attacks but also with making right choices while buying groceries and eating out in restaurants.

Let's take a closer look on what this book has to offer:

A - The Research

This part of the book educates you not only about the Migraine disease itself but other various types of Migraines too. It covers the various kinds of Migraines one can suffer from, their possible causes and triggers. It also helps one in distinguishing the difference between normal headaches and real Migraine attacks. If you are a woman, this section is a must read as it will help you understand why Migraines are so common in woman.

Overall, this part of the book is a must read if you want to know what you are dealing with.

B – The Migraine Diet Guide

This part of the book educates you in great detail about the foods one should eat or avoid in order to keep the Migraine attacks away. This part of the book will unfold the foods from several food groups like **Breads, Cereals, Nuts and Seeds, Crackers, Chips, Cakes, Pies, Candies and Cookies, Drinks and Juices, Vegetables, Meat and Poultry, Fruits, Dairy Products, Sauces and Dips** and **Salad Dressings** that are best to eat and avoid if someone has Migraine problem. Each food group covered in this book has been carefully selected to make sure that foods consumed by people every day are covered entirely.

This section makes sure that the person who needs to be on Migraine diet is well-versed with the required dietary information and guidelines to live a healthy and Migraine free life.

Also Includes: Migraine Free Grocery Shopping List, Eating out Tips & Guidelines and Easy to Follow Self Help Measures

---

This additional part of the book is a must read for people suffering from Migraine attacks as it will cover the best possible **Grocery Shopping List** which you can use while buying your groceries, **Eating out Tips and Guidelines** which you can easily follow while eating out in restaurants to avoid further Migraine attacks and various easy to follow **Self Help Measures** for a complete Migraine Free life.

1

Understanding Migraine Disease

WHAT IS MIGRAINE?

A normal headache tends to go away with the resolution of a problem, sufficient rest, or appropriate medications. A migraine headache, however, refuses to do the same. In fact, it may last for anywhere between four to 72 hours.

You will be able to comprehend the difference, when you observe one side of your head throbbing with excruciating pain. This is why the Greeks categorized this kind of headache as "**hemikrania**," which literally means 'half of the head'. In case, the pain spreads over the entire cranium (skull), it may become tremendously difficult to bear. What makes it worse is the fact that you may experience nausea and vomiting, blurring of vision, and tingling sensations in the arms and legs too.

At the same time, your eyes are prone towards hypersensitivity to light. As a result, they tend to vacillate between the appearance of dark spots and flashes of light. Obviously, your head and eyes will desire refuge in a darkened room. Similarly, you begin to feel irked by loud sounds in your vicinity. Therefore, you may exhibit signs of irritability and moodiness. It follows that you will experience depression and anxiety; both will not permit you to eat, sleep, or work.

Above all, if you end up feeling too stressed, you are not going to find it easy to express yourself or be clear in speech. Thus, in this state of confusion, all you can hope and pray for, is quick relief from this debilitating condition.

UNDERLYING CAUSES

Surprisingly, no scientist has been able to pinpoint the exact cause of migraine disease. Obviously, scientifically approved methods and suitable equipment have been brought into play for every academic study. It is just that these studies have not been able to provide readymade answers yet.

Nevertheless, experts agree on a few things. They suggest that migraine disease is the outcome of a combination of genetic and environmental factors. They often focus on hormonal changes, chemical alterations within the brain, link between abnormal nerves and alterations of blood flow within blood vessels, etc. Even physicians tend to mistake them for tension headaches or sinus headaches at times, thereby resulting in further confusion for the patient. Not only adults, but also children may remain undiagnosed for years and years.

Since the causative factors are not clear, migraine headaches are the focus of academic debates, examinations and research even today, because numerous people across the world continue to suffer from this disease. Yes, the statistics may amaze you. In the U.S. alone, over 12% (36 million) of the population (men, women and children) suffers from migraine attacks. The patient may be as young as 10 or 15 years old; he/she may be middle-aged, that is, between 40 and 55 years old. Regardless, the peak years for falling prey to this disease lie between 25 and 55. Children often inherit the condition from their parents (40% chances, if one parent is stricken; 90% chances, if both parents are sufferers).

Just imagine; migraine disease seems to affect more people than asthma and diabetes combined do!

2

The Various Types of Migraine

Rarely does a migraine headache occur without warning; you just have to be alert enough to the unusual signs. To illustrate, you will become aware of the onset of a migraine attack if you are lucky enough to experience an 'aura.' Should you feel this aura before the attack, it will mean that you are experiencing a classic migraine headache. Around 15% to 20% of victims around the world suffer this kind of migraine disease.

MIGRAINE ATTACK WITH AN AURA

Now, do not be under the mistaken impression that this term refers to something glamorous or ethereal! No, indeed, it does not; it merely refers to something scientific or physiological in nature. Your vision may seem to have become distorted, just an hour or so before you are actually attacked by a migraine headache. There seem to be bright lights or flashing dots dancing in front of your eyes. Sometimes, it may seem as if you can only visualize dark spots or blind spots in front of you. Alternatively, you may feel that you have lost your sight completely. Then again, everything may appear jagged or wavy.

Your eyes are not the only senses to send out warning signals, however. Your other senses get into the act too. For instance, you may experience a 'funny feeling' or just feel uneasy. You may not be able to explain it in so many words. Then again, you may believe that you are surrounded by strange odors, or smells different from the ordinary. Even the taste of food or the touch of something may feel unusual. Sometimes, there is a ringing in your ears; it is known as **tinnitus**.

Whatever is the case, the 'aura' tends to last anywhere between 15 minutes and one hour. An aura may even be felt soon after the onset of a migraine attack or during the attack itself. Whatever is the case, you will be prepared for a massive headache.

MIGRAINE ATTACK WITHOUT AN AURA

Yes, of course. This is known as a **common migraine headache**. If you experience this kind of an attack, you may count yourself amongst the majority. Around 85% or more sufferers around the world tend to experience migraine disease without an aura. Regardless of the absence of an aura, you may feel fatigued, anxious, or depressed without a valid reason at times. Such feelings come to the fore just a few hours prior to the onset of an excruciatingly painful headache.

On the other hand, you may experience a sudden craving for sweets. Then again, you may feel tremendously sleepy or thirsty, again without a plausible reason. Whatever kinds of signs come to the fore, you may expect to suffer for at least 72 hours. All this is fine, but you are still confused about recognizing the onset of a migraine attack, since you do not experience an aura beforehand, aren't you?

PHASES OF MIGRAINE ATTACKS

Well, you could follow the advice of experts, who suggest that people like you should learn to recognize the following three distinct phases associated with your unique kind of headache. Note that they occur only in common migraine headaches.

Prodrome

The first phase is known as **"prodrome"** or the **"pre-headache"** stage. It is possible to experience this phase a few hours prior, or even a few days prior, to the actual attack. For instance, you may feel rather astonished by your sudden cravings for all kinds of foodstuffs. Then again, your muscles seem to go all stiff, or your moods keep changing all the time without any warning. There may be other signs too, different from the ordinary, which suggest that you are about to experience a massive headache.

Headache

The second phase is known as the **"headache"** phase, wherein you experience debilitating pain not only in the cranial region, but also in the entire body. You have fallen prey to a migraine attack.

Postdrome

The last phase is the **"postdrome"** stage, wherein you feel extremely fatigued. Alternatively, you may feel like you are having a hangover.

Sometimes, you may bypass the second phase, that is, the "headache" phase. You may experience only the first and third phases. Regardless the kind of headache, it will still be categorized as migraine disease by doctors. They address this malady as **'silent'** migraine or **'acephalgic'** migraine, since the second stage is absent. Of course, the usual symptoms of migraine disease are the same amongst all patients, regardless of whether they experience an aura or not.

MULTIPLE KINDS OF MIGRAINES

Amazingly, you may suffer from multiple kinds of migraines, especially if you are prone towards experiencing an aura prior to an attack. Thankfully, 'multiple' suffering is a rare occurrence.

Retinal Migraine

In certain instances, vision may seem to be partially, completely, or temporarily lost in one eye. This is accompanied by a dull ache behind the eye (Retinal region). The ache gradually spreads along the entire skull region. This is referred to as Retinal migraine.

Ophthalmoplegic Migraine

Alternatively, you may experience a painful ache around the entire eye. This is known as **Ophthalmoplegic migraine** (ophthalmic = relating to eye; plegia = paralysis). The muscles in the region of this eye appear to be paralyzed too. Do not take this situation lightly, for the nerves in the region behind this eye are being pressurized. You do not wish to suffer a burst blood vessel or aneurysm (weakening and widening of artery wall); consult a doctor immediately.

A few other symptoms of this disease are visible changes in vision, occurrence of double vision, or a droopy eyelid.

Hemiplegic Migraine

Sometimes, you may fall victim to Hemiplegic migraine (partial paralysis). In this case, one side of your body experiences temporary paralysis, sensory changes, or nerve changes. As a result, you may feel dizzy or numb, albeit temporarily. Even your vision seems to be distorted.

Familiar Hemiplegic Migraine

In case, your migraine disease is linked to your genes, you could be suffering from Familiar Hemiplegic migraine. As a result, your headache tends to last for five or ten days, accompanied by drowsiness, confusion and one-sided paralysis.

You may even slip into a temporary coma, prompting the physician to mistake your condition for epilepsy.

Basilar Artery Migraine

Then again, you may suffer from basilar artery migraine (supplies blood to some parts of your brain and inner ear). In this case, you may experience sudden symptoms of confusion, dizziness, vomiting, ringing in the ears, loss of balance, or an inability to express yourself lucidly. They appear just before your headache begins. The pain is extremely severe at the back of the head. This kind of migraine is believed to affect young women, who are experiencing hormonal changes within their bodies.

Status Migrainosus

Status migrainosus (status = the state you are in at a particular time; migrainosus = headache that lasts beyond 72 hours) is the worst kind of malady that you can suffer. It can be extremely debilitating, even requiring immediate hospitalization at times. The nausea and pain accompanying the onset of this kind of migraine are terribly traumatic and intense. The onset may be attributed to the consumption or sudden withdrawal of specific medications.

Abdominal Migraine

If your child experiences recurring abdominal pain, accompanied by sudden loss of appetite, vomiting and nausea, he/she could be suffering from abdominal migraine. This attack tends to last anywhere between 1 and 72 hours.

Menstrual Migraine

Similarly, if you are a woman, who experiences intense headaches two days prior to beginning your menstrual period or two days after your menstrual period ends, you could be suffering from menstrual migraine. This kind of migraine attack is visible only during your monthly periods.

3

The Headaches vs. Real Migraine Attacks

Even with all your informative knowledge and awareness, it may be difficult to differentiate between an ordinary headache and migraine disease, sometimes. Here are some tips to help you identify each one.

THE ORDINARY HEADACHE

Let us suppose that you are experiencing some stress at your workplace, or beset by mild issues in the domestic arena. Too much of thinking about resolutions to pending problems can lead to a kind of aching pressure in your head region. Your forehead or temples seem to be pulsating more than other areas do. At other times, the neck region seems stiff and tense. Yet, the pain varies from mild to moderate; it rarely becomes intense. Furthermore, the pain is felt on both sides of your head; it is never one-sided. These symptoms indicate that you are suffering from a mild or moderate tension headache, which can be resolved easily.

Even stresses and strains involving muscles may usher in a severe headache. Although this kind of a headache rarely lasts over 30 minutes or an hour, it may stretch to a week because you refuse to let go off your thoughts or remain emotionally weak all the time. The duration may cause an inexperienced physician to conclude that you have migraine disease.

Similarly, you may be prone to sinus infections, especially when the climate changes. This will result in a sinus headache. Apart from the throbbing pain in your head, you will exhibit symptoms of cough and congestion, fever, and a stuffy nose. Even your face experiences pain and pressure. The symptoms are very similar to migraine disease; doctors can become confused.

A cluster headache is witnessed only one side of your head. The headache is accompanied by watery eyes, nasal congestion and a runny nose. Again, it may be related to changes in climate, or even allergies. Regardless, the one-sided pain is definitely not as severe as that experienced during a migraine attack.

Regardless of the kind of headache that you have, it is easily treatable. For instance, analgesics like aspirin, acetaminophen, or ibuprofen should suffice to take care of tension headaches. They are over-the-counter drugs. As for sinus headaches and cluster headaches, you may opt for prescribed drugs handed out by your family physician.

Of course, it would be good to avoid addiction to pills, and go in for relaxation techniques instead. You may request a professional for help with relaxation exercises, or even neck-stretching exercises. Simple yoga and meditation can go a long way in calming a stressed mind. Then again, request someone to massage your temples, forehead, or the back of your neck, for some time. This will reduce the tension in the muscles.

If possible, go in for the application of warm compresses on the affected region. Alternatively, just take a hot shower, play some soothing music, and rest. A brisk walk in the fresh air, spending some time on your favorite hobby, consultations with close friends, etc. are great options too. Whatever is the case, you can always find a suitable remedy to get rid of a normal headache.

THE MIGRAINE

As stated several times already, the pain experienced during a migraine attack is intensely severe in nature. You may even feel like banging your head against a wall, just to be rid of this tremendous trauma! It is as if your head is pulsating or pounding vigorously. What makes it worse is the fact that the ache is only on one side of the head.

Over time, the pain may spread across the entire head region. At the same time, it is possible to have a migraine attack on both sides of your head. However, this is not a common occurrence. Any kind of physical activity or exertion only serves to worsen the pain. In fact, concentrating on any kind of task will seem very difficult.

The beginning of a headache is not the only thing that causes you so much of misery; other symptoms may make an appearance too, especially a couple of days prior to the actual onset of severe migraine. For instance, your senses of touch, taste and smell seem to have gone all haywire. Nothing appears appropriate to your skin, tongue, or nose; everything seems different from the ordinary. In fact, strong odors tend to cause you a lot of discomfort. You may feel nauseous, or give in to bouts of vomiting.

Paradoxically, you may even feel the need for experimenting with varied foodstuffs. This kind of experimentation can lead to constipation at times. Your moods can undergo all kinds of changes, wherein you begin to feel depressed, anxious and irritated, all at the same time. This is because you tend to be slightly confused, and feel unable to think clearly. You may even find it difficult to put your thoughts into words; there is no clarity with language.

As if this is not enough, you begin to have trouble with body balance too. Photophobia (excessive sensitivity to light) and phonophobia (excessive sensitivity to sound) are also common. This hypersensitivity to light can make you feel as if dark spots and flashing lights are all around the eye near the migraine headache. Similarly, your ear seems to ache all the time. A tingling sensation is felt in the arms and legs. Surprisingly, even with all these disturbances, you tend to feel sleepy most of the time, giving in to frequent bouts of yawning. Above all, your neck may feel stiff and tense.

Please note; it is not necessary for any patient to experience every single symptom associated with migraine headache. Every person's constitution is different. Only the excruciatingly painful headache is common amongst all. As for the presence or absence of an aura, only the doctor will be able to help you differentiate, in alignment with your signs and symptoms.

You would be well advised not to purchase over-the-counter medications for treating your migraine disease. Yes, there are specific medicines for treating nausea, wonderful non-steroidal anti-inflammatory drugs for dealing with pain, healthy anti-depressants, safe medications for lowering high blood pressure, etc. However, it would not do to take migraine headaches lightly, since they are related to alterations within the brain and nerves.

Then again, you must remember that your malady is a frequent visitor in your life. Would it not be better to find sensible relaxation techniques for dealing with unwanted stress? You could even go in for dietary changes, avoiding foodstuffs that actually trigger headaches. Just keep in mind that professional help is always available; take advantage of it.

4

The Causes and Triggers of Migraine

Even the most scientifically inclined experts across the globe have never been able to comprehend the exact causes of migraine attacks that well. At best, they can offer varied theories.

THE CORTICAL SPREADING DEPRESSION (CSD) THEORY

The Cortical Spreading Depression (CSD) theory advocates that migraine disease may be related to malfunctioning of the brain, just as angina is associated with the inappropriate functioning of the heart. According to this theory, there may be a sudden, local and transient suppression (termed as 'depression' in the scientific world) of the electrical activity that takes place within the cortex region (cortical) of your brain. This suppression gradually spreads across the entire region, giving rise to symptoms of an impending migraine attack.

This theory was publicized in 1994 by Aristides A. P. Leao, and has been tested several times ever since. Thus, there is positive confirmation of the CSD theory, but its actual role in the onset of migraine disease is still in doubt; further studies are required. This is because healthcare providers, who believed in the CSD theory, had attempted to treat migraine patients with a drug (Tonabersat) to block the occurrence or enhancement of CSD. However, the drug failed to offer any kind of relief; people continued to suffer.

THE VASCULAR THEORY

Academicians then tried to explore another theory known as the **vascular theory**. This theory suggests that blood flow within your brain becomes abnormal, due to the widening of the blood vessels around the brain. However, there is no relevant explanation for why this should happen.

A third theory suggests that alterations may take place in the brainstem (the part of the brain connecting with the spinal cord at the back of the neck). These alterations may be attributed to a drop in serotonin levels. Known as the "**happy**" chemical, Serotonin is manufactured in your brain and intestines. It ensures that your moods remain well balanced, controls pain, regulates social behavior, acts as a messenger for your nervous system, etc.

You can well imagine the impact on your mind and body, if Serotonin levels drop suddenly. Within the brain itself, the drop may prompt the trigeminal system (sensory nerves related to 'pain') to release some chemicals of its own. When these chemicals travel to the brainstem, they result in excruciatingly painful headaches.

Whatever is the case, the exact causes of migraine disease have yet to be determined. If environmental factors are to be considered, they may relate to alterations in the blood flow, unusual chemical reactions, or malfunction of nerves. If genetic factors are to be considered, the trauma is passed on from generation to generation naturally.

WHAT TRIGGERS IT?

Is it possible to identify the triggers of migraine attacks, even if the causes are vague? Yes, it is entirely possible to take note of possible triggers that result in so much of trauma.

Family History

To begin with, check out your family history. Does one parent suffer from migraine attacks? It is possible for both parents to be patients too. If your answer is in the affirmative, you stand a good chance of inheriting migraine disease. This should not come as a surprise, for several diseases are inherited from immediate family or past generations.

Age is no barrier to migraine attacks. You may become a victim anytime during childhood, adolescence, young adulthood, or late adulthood. When you experience your first attack, you may expect the disease to become chronic later on.

Food

Since you live in the 21st century with all its temptations, especially heavenly smelling and delicious-tasting junk foods, you may be placing yourself at high risk for migraine disease. Yes, foods stuffed with salt, as well as processed foods are likely to trigger migraine attacks, especially if you love to gorge on them. Some people are not comfortable with aged cheeses. You will have to take note of your dietary habits and cravings, to discover what invites migraine headaches.

Alternatively, your constitution may be sensitive to specific food additives. For instance, a preservative like monosodium glutamate (Ajinomoto, tasting powder, etc.) or a sweetener like aspartame (Equal, NutraSweet, etc.) may trigger a migraine headache. Certain preservatives or sweeteners are found in many foodstuffs, especially those that have to be on the shelves for a long time.

Caffeine & Alcohol

Are you addicted to caffeinated beverages or alcoholic drinks? If you do not place a limit on the amounts that you consume, you are bound to fall prey to migraine disease. Instead of relaxing your mind, these beverages will stress it excessively. Sometimes, your stomach feels heavily filled with liquids, or your appetite becomes weak. As a result, you refuse to eat sufficient quantities of food at the right mealtimes. Fasting, whether voluntarily or involuntarily, can lead to migraine attacks.

Sleep & Rest Patterns

It is possible that your normal waking-and-sleeping patterns become disturbed due to shifts in work timings, jet lag, etc. Then again, you may be such a workaholic that you do not pay much attention to obtaining sufficient rest and sleep. Of course, a couple of days without adequate sleep may merely lead to severe headache.

However, if you continue to stress your mind and body for a long time, you are bound to become a target of migraine disease. Paradoxically, even too much of sleep can lead to heaviness and pain in the head. It all depends upon how your constitution handles your altering sleep-wake patterns.

Environmental

In case, you are an extremely sensitive person, changes in the environment, such as sudden weather changes, drop or rise in barometric pressure, etc., may bother you immensely. Then again, you may dislike loud sounds and bright lights intensely. The sounds emanating from moving traffic, blaring speakers, the harsh glare of the sun, brilliant light bulbs, etc. can induce migraine headaches.

At times, unusual odours may trouble you. Such odours include smells emanating from paint thinners, perfumes, second-hand smoke, and so on. You have to be careful about medications and therapies too. For instance, vasodilators (nitroglycerin), oral contraceptives, estrogen replacement therapy, etc. may induce and aggravate migraine headaches. If you are a woman, take note of your hormonal changes with the aid of a doctor. They induce migraines at times.

Physical

Surprisingly, excessive physical exertion, including intense sexual activity, can also trigger a migraine attack. You expect to sleep peacefully after being so active, but you tend to stay awake with an aching head!

Psychological

Of course, the biggest culprit is stress. You are bound to find all kinds of stressors at home, in the workplace, and in the community. It may not be possible for you to remain positive all the time. As soon as your spirit sinks too low, your head begins to throb with tension. Gradually, you become a patient of migraine disease.

5

Women and Migraines

You may feel astonished to know that women are more susceptible to migraine attacks than men are. Age does not matter, for migraine disease can strike any time. Nonetheless, girls become more vulnerable once they attain puberty. Boys are at higher risk during childhood. According to the latest statistics, more than 27 million American women are victims of migraine disease today.

WHY IS THIS SO?

This is because women like you tend to undergo diverse hormonal changes throughout their lives. Based upon individual constitution, you may experience one, or even several migraine attacks every month.

Let us suppose that you are going in for birth control pills, since it is a very popular form of hormonal contraception. In case, you have a family history of migraine disease, you may experience your first attack when you begin taking the pills. In case, you are already prone to migraine headaches, hormonal contraception (administered orally, via a patch, through injections, or into the vagina) may serve to enhance the pain, reduce it, or have no effect on the pain at all. Therefore, please consult a physician before choosing the mode of hormonal contraception.

Then again, there is menstrual migraine. You may experience severe headaches two days prior to the onset of your cycle, or for three consecutive days at the end of the cycle. This kind of migraine is rather difficult to treat, since the severity, symptoms, duration and response to medications vary from individual to individual. Hormonal fluctuations (related to estrogen) only serve to make the condition worse. In case, you do not respond well to medications, the doctor may advise hormonal contraceptives as an alternative. They either eliminate your menstrual periods, or reduce their frequency.

Now, you could be planning a pregnancy, or may be already pregnant. With regard to the former, strong medications may not permit you to conceive. With regard to the latter, the fetus within your womb may be harmed. Regardless, it is heartening to note that over 60% of sufferers do find their headaches improving during the first trimester of pregnancy. Over 75% discover that the disease either improves or completely disappears during the next two trimesters. On the negative side, a significant lot find their migraine disease worsening, or remaining unaffected.

DURING AND AFTER MENOPAUSE

You will be able to heave a sigh of relief, since your hormones stop fluctuating, along with the cessation of your menstrual cycles. Your headaches improve. If you are lucky, the migraine disease will disappear completely. Thereafter, you need not worry. In case, you have reached menopause or beyond without experiencing migraine disease, you may consider yourself lucky! Rarely does this malady strike a woman over 60 or 65 years of age.

6

The Diet Guide for Migraine Disease

Ah, yes, it is the age of the "body beautiful!" Naturally, you are so eager to look perfect that you rarely spare a thought for the ill effects that might accrue from your unhealthy eating habits or other actions. One negative outcome, amongst several others, is the onset of migraine disease.

If I need to tell you in short then I would suggest you to please keep your body and skin well hydrated, by drinking at least 8 to 10 glasses of water each day. If you dislike plain water, go in for decaffeinated coffee, fat-free milk or herbal tea sometimes.

Similarly, add Riboflavin (B2) supplement and foods containing omega-3 fatty acids (olive oil, canola oil, wild salmon, fatty fish, etc.) to your diet. Magnesium-rich foods (whole grains, Swiss chard, sweet potatoes, sunflower seeds, spinach, brown rice, white potatoes, quinoa and fresh amaranth) are splendid for reduction and prevention of all types of migraines.

FOOD ADDITIVES TO AVOID

You have learned that specific foods may behave like migraine triggers. It would be best to avoid them as much as possible. Let's now see what food additives make foods unsafe for migraine.

- **Monosodium glutamate (MSG)** is a favorite flavor enhancer, which is added to fermented, pickled, or marinated foodstuffs. You might try to reduce your consumption of such foods. MSG is also an integral ingredient of frozen foods, canned vegetables, processed foods, canned soups and seasonings. You cannot give up everything that you like; just try to stay within safe limits of consumption.

- **Tyramine**: Then again, aged cheeses, such as cheddar, blue cheese and Parmesan contain a monoamine, known as **Tyramine**. This is definitely a migraine trigger. The same ingredient is found in smoked fish, onions and cured sausages as well. Avoid red wine, as it increases migraine attacks. Even white wine and beer should not be consumed heavily. They contain Tyramine.

- **Sodium nitrate**: Ah, yes, you love hot dogs, don't you? Well, Tyramine and sodium nitrate (preservative) are integral ingredients of varied brands of hot dogs. The same ingredients are also found in bacon, pepperoni, sausage, salami and luncheon meat.

■ **Aspartame**: Like many people, you may opt for diet sodas, low-calorie treats and snack foods, believing that they will aid with weight management. Do note that an artificial sweetener called **aspartame** is found in these beverages and foods. The sweetener is a migraine trigger.

Caffeinated products, beverages, sodas, energy drinks and chocolates are marvelous for enhancing alertness and keeping pain in control, provided they are consumed in small amounts. Otherwise, they may serve to increase your pain, irksomeness, anxiety and insomnia. If you are addicted to them, your body may experience chemical intolerance. Sudden withdrawal, on the other hand, will bring on a migraine attack.

SUGAR AND MIGRAINE RELATION

Similar to a machine, your body needs fuel (energy) in order to function well throughout the day. This fuel is obtained from foodstuffs containing carbohydrates. Once these carbohydrates enter your digestive tract, they are converted into glucose through various processes. Of course, the ability to supply energy remains intact, whatever form the carbohydrates take. Your bloodstream supplies this glucose to various parts of your body, including the brain.

Your brain is the 'master controller' of your body. Therefore, you can well imagine how much of glucose it requires throughout the day if it has to achieve peak performance. The entire process, that is, digestion, distribution and absorption, takes around three to four hours to be completed. At this time, you find it easy to perform all your tasks efficiently.

However, the fuel cannot last forever; it is bound to deplete. You will realize it when you begin to feel less energetic or weak. Your body is demanding a fresh batch of glucose via food. This is precisely why medical experts suggest that you adhere to four-hourly gaps between meals during the day. The time gap between dinner and breakfast should not go beyond 12 hours.

- Despite knowing this, you may become so involved in domestic chores, office work, or other activities, that you forget all about your hungry stomach.

- Alternatively, you may have decided to go on a rigorous diet or fast. Naturally, you are bound to skip meals or eat insufficient amounts of food.

- Sometimes, you are overenthusiastic about your morning exercises, quite forgetting that you have been fasting all night.

- If you are fond of sweets, confectionaries, or foodstuffs stuffed with artificial sugars, your bloodstream is bound to find itself suddenly burdened with excess glucose. This cannot be allowed to happen. Therefore, your pancreas takes charge and begins to release more insulin. It is as if insulin is at one end of a seesaw, while glucose is at the other end. The tussle takes its toll, and your blood-glucose levels fall sharply.

■ In case, you are a diabetic, you may inject too much insulin into your body at times. This can cause a drop in glucose levels.

Medical experts term this condition as Hypoglycemia. You will recognize the condition when you begin to experience some, or all of these symptoms – nausea, dizziness, headache, excessive yawning, sweating, fall in body temperature, pallor, craving for sugary stuff, mood changes and confusion. Obviously, your brain is the culprit. Its craving for glucose prompts more blood to flow into it, and with greater speed. Even the blood vessels dilate, thereby leading to enhanced nerve sensitivity and pain. You are definitely heading for a severe migraine attack.

Keeping the blood sugar levels stable

In actuality, your body is well equipped to maintain balanced blood-sugar levels. It has two hormones known as **glucagon** and insulin to help it. Whenever the glucose levels drop, glucagon ensures that they get back on track. Whenever the glucose levels rise, insulin goes into its balancing act. It helps that both these hormones are rapid in action. An imbalance occurs only when you interfere with your body's natural functioning via your unhealthy lifestyle. Regardless, do not despair. There are ways to stabilize your blood-glucose levels and avoid migraine attacks.

■ For instance, it would be good to create a dietary regimen that includes foodstuffs with low glycemic index (GI). You may opt for dairy products (custard, milk and yoghurt), fruits (strawberries, peaches, grapes, oranges and plums), snacks (oatmeal crackers, nuts, hummus and corn chips), pulses (lentils, kidney beans, black eyed beans and chick peas), vegetables (carrots, frozen peas, broccoli and sweet corn), or whole grain foods (wholegrain bread, wheat pasta and brown rice). They release the carbohydrate components within them in a slow manner. This allows for proper and healthy digestion and assimilation within your body. Glucose levels remain normal.

■ Pleasure-awarding substances or quick energy boosters like white bread, chips, watermelon, sugary foods, dates, sweetened breakfast cereals and baked potatoes fall into the high glycemic index category. You would do well to have a healthy mix of nutritious foods (80%) and 'pleasure' (20%) foods. Do not become obsessed with health concerns and place too many restrictions on yourself.

■ Experiment with alternatives. For instance, you might combine peanut butter and whole meal toast, thereby providing your body with the required amounts of protein, fats and carbohydrates. Substitute biscuits and chocolates with raisins and nuts. Do ensure that your meals have sufficient fiber in them, as it aids in healthy digestion and prevents the advent of constipation.

■ Do not skip breakfast at any cost. It is the most essential meal of the day. Eat little if you want to, but eat!

■ Instead of going in for a couple or more of large meals per day, go in for five small meals. Space them out, such that you might eat little, but oftener. Your stomach will be grateful for your thoughtfulness in permitting it to work slowly and harmoniously.

- Please stay away from excessively cold or hot beverages. Consume them at room temperature.

- In case, you wish to engage in mild or moderate exercise, do so a couple of hours after eating. Rigorous activity may warrant a three-hour gap. You may consume glucose sweets prior to exercising, just to grant yourself more energy.

- It is essential to consume water before, during and after physical activities. You lose body fluids through sweating; they have to be replaced quickly. You could use isotonic (mixture of glucose and mineral salts) drinks instead of water.

- Do you wake up in the middle of the night with an agonizing headache? Consume a protein snack prior to going to sleep.

MIGRAINE SAFE AND UN-SAFE FOODS BY CATEGORY

Food groups may be categorized as safe or unsafe based upon the form in which they are consumed.

Bread

It is one of the easiest things to purchase and consume, especially when you are in a hurry.

Safe - Ensure that you buy wheat, rye, zucchini, pumpernickel or white bread from reputable stores only. Yeast-based breads should be around 24 hours old. Then again, you may opt for bagels (filled with sesame seeds or plain) or English muffins.

Unsafe – Consume limited quantities of breads containing cheese, nuts, chocolate, or raisins. Bagels containing dried cranberries or blueberries, fresh donuts, freshly baked bread (whether bought from a bakery or made at home) fresh breakfast Danish and pizza are not good for your health either.

Cereals

Anything prepared from grains is viewed as an ideal breakfast recipe. Nevertheless, it always pays to be careful.

Safe – You are welcome to purchase most of the reputed brands advertised in the marketplace.

Unsafe – Cereals containing coconuts, raisins, aspartame, chocolate, peanut butter, nuts, or dried fruits may appeal highly to your taste buds, but still deemed as unhealthy.

Nuts and Seeds

You may feel that they have little value, apart from garnishing a particular dish. However, they are extremely nutritious, even if consumed in minimal amounts.

Safe – Popcorn is great as a teatime snack, but only if it is prepared at home and consumed without additional flavors. As for seeds, you may opt for poppy, pumpkin, sunflower (no natural flavor) or sesame.

Unsafe – Nuts are not good for migraine patients. Even butters (including peanut butter) are to be sidelined. Popcorn that has come out from the microwave oven or garnished with Cheddar cheese, is a big "No-No." Finally, even if you adore them, avoid consuming almond extract or coconut.

Crackers

Like everybody else, you may love to snack on crackers. However, are all crackers healthy?

Safe – There are several brands available at stores. Select those that are unflavored.

Unsafe – Try to keep away from flavored varieties, as well as cheese crackers.

Chips

You can carry them everywhere. They are generally so delicious that it is hard to keep track of your consumption!

Safe – Well, you might be wise to adhere to Herr's salt and vinegar chips, all kinds of plain potato chips, Frito's corn chips, all kinds of plain pretzels and Tostitos 100% corn chips.

Unsafe – As a migraine sufferer, you had best keep away from seasoned chips like jalapeno, Pringles, Doritos Nacho, etc. similarly, stay away from pretzels that have been seasoned with mustard, garlic, honey, etc. Soft pretzels are not good either.

Cakes, Pies, Candies and Cookies

Sugary foodstuffs and confectionaries have never been considered as nutritious, especially if consumed frequently.

Safe – You will be happy to know that your migraine disease will not be affected by the consumption of shortbread cookies, oatmeal cookies without raisins, store-bought apple pies (no lemon juice in them), blueberry pies (store-bought and no lemon juice), rice pudding minus raisins, strawberry wafers, vanilla wafers, white chocolate, cinnamon swirl cakes, or vanilla cakes.

Unsafe – Your migraine will become more painful if you gorge on coconut, nuts, aspartame-containing products (advertised as sugar-free or diet products), chocolate candy, almond extract, chocolate, peanut butter, lemon juice, buttermilk, lemon extract, sour cream, or dried fruit.

Drinks and Juices

Refreshing beverages may be consumed at any time of the day or night.

Safe – Decaffeinated (naturally) tea and coffee are welcome. Additionally, you may drink white milk, chamomile tea (caffeine-free), vodka and fruit juices (grape, pear, apricot, apple and cranberry). Caffeine-free colas and beers are fine too.

Unsafe – Do not become addicted to diet sodas containing saccharin or aspartame, strong alcoholic beverages, caffeinated teas and coffees, chocolate milk, hot chocolate, caffeinated root beer, beer, wine, colas, champagne, lemon lime soda, orange soda, Mountain Dew, or coffee substitutes.

Vegetables

Astonishingly, your migraine disease does not believe in the positive benefits of some vegetables.

Safe – You have a wide choice from amongst carrots, cauliflower, garlic, fresh potatoes, zucchini, turnips, frozen peas, canned peas, corn, spring onions, plain rice, Brussels' sprouts, shallots, peppers, eggplant, okra, yams, asparagus, preservative-free bagged lettuce, leeks, frozen mashed potatoes (some kinds), artichokes, broccoli, chick peas, string beans, corn, squash, red beets, mushrooms and some beans.

Unsafe – You must keep away from navy beans, instant mashed potatoes, onions, lentils, broad Italian beans, sauerkraut, fava beans, pea pods and lima beans.

Meat and Poultry

Safe – You are allowed to have fish, fresh chicken, pork, veal, turkey, lamb and beef. Ensure that broth or tenderizer has not been injected into the meat. Sausages possessing no natural flavors, MSG or onion, may be consumed safely.

Unsafe – Avoid marinated meat, barbequed chicken, beef liver, chicken liver, readymade hot wings, canned tuna containing broth, breaded meat or chicken patties, seasoned chicken, ham containing nitrites, hot dogs, canned soups, anchovies, most lunchmeats, spam and readymade meals with meat or noodles.

Fruits

Fruits and fruit juices are marvellous for your health, but not all of them.

Safe – Watermelon, strawberries, blackberries, blueberries, grapes, cherries, peaches, honeydew melon, apples, kiwi, peaches, pears, mangoes, apricots, cantaloupes and nectarines. Make sure that the fruits are fresh.

Unsafe – Sulfite-preserved dried fruits, lemons, raisins, Clementine's, bananas, pineapples, raspberries, limes, dates, avocados, grapefruit, tangerines, oranges, papayas, passion fruit, plums and figs.

Dairy Products

You may have to stay away from quite a few favorites.

Safe – Apart from white milk, you may consume various kinds of cheeses (ricotta, Deli American, cottage, cream and American with jalapeno peppers).

Unsafe – Chocolate milk (contains caffeine), aged cheeses (Monterey Jack, Swiss, Cheddar and Colby), pizza, Brie, mozzarella cheese, yoghurt, sour cream, hot pockets and buttermilk, are to be avoided.

Sauces and Dips

Safe – Home-made stuff.

Unsafe – Purchased stuff contains MSG or onions. Keep away from tomato sauce, guacamole, mustard dips, chips dips, mustard dips, gravy, salsa and barbeque sauce.

Salad Dressing

Safe – Distilled white vinegar and any oil are healthy.

Unsafe – Avoid bottled dressings, for they contain natural flavors, MSG, vinegar (not white), grated cheese, onion powder, or onion.

7

The Recommended Grocery Shopping List

Shopping for groceries can prove to be quite a chore for a migraine patient. There are so many things to remember. The detailed list may prove helpful.

Cereals

You may begin the day with cornflakes, shredded wheat, Cheerios, Uncle Sam, Grape Nuts, Frosted Flakes, Life, or Golden Grahams.

Beverages

It is quite difficult to give up your morning cup of coffee or tea entirely, isn't it? Do not worry, for equally aromatic substitutes are available. The best one is chamomile herb tea from Celestial Seasonings. If you promise to consume only a couple of cups a day, you might try naturally decaffeinated green tea from Lipton or naturally decaffeinated instant coffee offered by Taster's Choice. It would be best to stay away from naturally decaffeinated drip coffee, unless you plan to drink it rarely.

Soda

Go in for diet root beer and black cherry, mug root beer, black cherry, Waist Watcher's cola, caffeine-free Pepsi or Coke, and Diet Rite cola. These products contain no aspartame or caffeine. Purchase bottled water whenever you are eating out.

Vegetables

Look out for baked potatoes, fresh baby carrots, frozen Brussels' Sprouts, fresh tomatoes, frozen broccoli and celery. As for lettuce, do not purchase something that is displayed in a case. The product may contain sulfite. Instead, request for Fresh Express bagged lettuce. It contains no preservatives.

In case, you wish to buy canned tomato products, look for the brand called **Contadina**. This company offers crushed tomatoes in puree, tomato paste and diced tomatoes. None of them contains the food additive, MSG. It is a common flavoring agent used by other brands. You may like to buy El Rio's refried beans. Rest assured that it is free of MSG or onions.

Fruits

One should not get tempted by tins of dried fruit. Manufacturers generally use sulfites to keep the fruit looking fresh. In the absence of this preservative, the fruits may turn brown in color. Some establishments like Mariani retain the fruit color with the aid of sulfur dioxide. This should be harmless. Nevertheless, it is safe to buy canned pears, canned peaches, strawberries, pears, grapes, apples and blueberries.

Seeds

Everyone knows that consumption of sunflower seeds is healthy. Well then, look for Here's How on the label. This company does not combine MSG with these seeds. Planters' Brand, on the other hand, uses MSG.

Cheese

Your best bet is Clearfield or Land-O-Lakes. The slices are of marvelous quality.

Breadcrumbs

Many breadcrumbs are laden with MSG. Kellogg's Cornflake crumbs are dependable and safe. Alternatively, you may just make some breadcrumbs at home.

Butter

You can make sunflower butter at home. Alternatively, you may purchase peanut butter from outside.

It is easy to make butter from sunflower seeds. To begin with, roast around 12 ounces of raw sunflower seeds (with hulls removed) at a temperature of 300 degrees. Seven to ten minutes of roasting should do the trick. Do not extend the time, for your butter will acquire a dry and burnt taste. Therefore, keep an eye on the clock. When you are through, place the seeds in a blender or food processor. Ensure that you obtain a fine powder. Now, add half-a-teaspoon of salt and one tablespoon of sugar to the powder. Pour half-a-cup of vegetable oil over the mixture. Use the blender/food processor to obtain a smooth paste. Your butter is ready to be stored in the refrigerator. The best thing is that the butter remains for a long time, without the taste or freshness being destroyed.

Oh, yes, if you wish to use mayonnaise instead of butter, do not go in for store purchases. If you have the time and patience, prepare it at home.

Jams

You might try blackberry jam prepared by Smucker's company. If you do not like its taste, you could always go back to grape, raspberry, or strawberry jam. However, blackberries can stimulate your palate, and leave it craving for more!

Fruit Juices

You may substitute your regular orange juice with Mango Peach. The product is manufactured by a company called **VS Splash**. Then again, the cranberry juice manufactured by Ocean Spray has a splendid taste. Furthermore, it is tough on the calories.

Soups

It would be best to avoid them as far as possible, for they contain preservatives and additives, which have a negative effect on migraines. Regardless, you may try Campbell's canned tomato soup occasionally.

Dairy Products

White milk and eggs may be consumed without fear.

Bagels

You cannot consume freshly made bagels, since they contain fresh yeast. They have to be stored for 24 hours before they may be eaten. Waiting for such a long time may prove rather frustrating. A better alternative would be to purchase Thomas's New York Style's plain bagels or bagels filled with sesame seeds. These large-sized bagels taste fresh and nice. They may be stored in the refrigerator.

Chips

Please avoid Pringles' products and flavored chips, if you do not wish to ruin your health. You may be interested to know that Pringles preserves dehydrated potato flakes with the help of bisulfate. This preservative ensures that the product does not lose its color during lengthy storage. You will not find this information on the label. It is the same for all mashed potato products stored in boxes. Instead of Pringles' products, go in for 100% white corn chips from Tostitos.

Cookies

If it is not possible to make cookies at home, you may opt for Keebler's Sandies Swirl Cinnamon Shortbread cookies. Some brands of crème wafers with a vanilla flavor are marvelous too. Do not go in for cookies prepared from buttermilk. They will aggravate your migraine.

Fish

Whenever you visit a departmental store, look for a gold and black can with Bumble Bee tuna written on it. This product does not contain hydrolyzed protein, soy protein, or vegetable broth. Therefore, it is safe for consumption.

Meat

In case, you want healthy chicken broth from cans, you are out of luck. The canned product contains onions and MSG. Additionally; there are no substitutes for this product. You have no choice, but to prepare it at home yourself. However, it is possible to purchase canned chicken, which does not contain MSG. Some manufacturers, including Sweet Sue, supply this product to stores. Similarly, you may be able to obtain canned chicken breast for making chicken salad.

With regard to lunchmeats, you may trust Carolina. This establishment supplies turkey breast coated with salt, and nothing more. You need not worry about the presence of MSG or nitrites.

It would be best to avoid tenderized meat, but Hatfield's products are an exception. Labeled as Simply Tender, these pork products are tenderized with the aid of lemon juice marinade, which is safe.

Dipping Mustard

The best purchase is Hot and Sweet from Bookbinders. The product contains white vinegar instead of MSG. This mustard is meant for pretzels.

Treats

The easiest way to treat self is to chew on dried caramels. Alternatively, you may go in for vanilla or strawberry ice creams. Breyer's is a good brand. Smucker's offers toppings in the form of caramel and frozen strawberries.

8

Eating Out Tips and Guidelines

It is true that there is no place like home, and there is no better meal than a home-cooked one. Yet, you do get tired of cooking your own meals or even eating what seems like the "same old stuff" day after day. Naturally, you get this urge to sample "outside" stuff sometimes. Viewed logically, this should not pose too much of a problem, since you are well aware of your limited food choices. The tips outlined below should serve to help you enjoy yourself without becoming unduly stressed.

■ Maybe, all that you want is a burger at a sit-down place. Do give clear instructions about how you wish your burger to be cooked and prepared. It should be devoid of onions, any kind of seasoning, or unseasoned fries.

- Then again, you may decide to eat at the renowned McDonald's restaurant. According to the experts, who also suffer from migraine as you do, you are sure to obtain whatever you want at McDonald's, if you word your requests properly. For instance, you may gorge on double burgers, fries and quarter pounders to your heart's content, since they are devoid of onions, MSG and seasoning. Do not touch the sauce, though. If you desire grilled chicken, you will have to check out the way it is prepared. You are welcome to end your meal with a strawberry or vanilla milkshake.

- Of course, McDonald's is only an example. You are bound to find several fast food restaurants in your locality offering similar menus. However, not all of them may be as accommodating towards their customers' special requests, as McDonald's is. It would be best to make a list of the ingredients you should avoid and keep it with you. Whether the restaurant is willing to accede to your request or not, you can always ask the waiter about recipes and preparations. Provide an explanation about your migraine disease, albeit briefly.

- As for restaurants and takeaways offering pizza and other kinds of Italian food, you would do well to forget about them. Pizza is made from fresh bread, which you must avoid at all costs. Onions seem to be an essential ingredient in the sauces on display. Even if you go in for mere salads, you have to be wary of their dressings. Unless they comprise of salt, pepper and plain oil, you would do well to leave them alone.

■ It is the same with Chinese food. You can never be sure of the ingredients, because these cooks tend to experiment with everything.

■ Suppose you plan to enter Subway shops. You may have a hard time finding something that suits your 'head,' not your palate. Their grilled chicken is generally seasoned with MSG. Then again, lunchmeats and fresh bread are their specialties, but you are forbidden to eat them. In case, you decide to go in for low-carbohydrate, veggie wraps, you will encounter another enemy of migraine disease, which is, soy protein. Even the products listed on the Atkins Diet, are dangerous for you.

■ You might try bagels made from yeast as an alternative to home-cooked food. However, the bagels are baked just ten minutes before they are served to customers. Therefore, purchase these fresh bagels, but do not consume them immediately. Bring them home and eat them a day (24 hours) later.

■ If you order steak at a fancy restaurant, ensure that it is neither seasoned nor tenderized.

In case, you wish to drink something, please carry your own soda bottle with you. Alternatively, you may carry some decaffeinated tea bags with you.

9

Best Self-help Measures for Migraine

Your physician may offer medications to tackle a migraine attack after it hits you. This individual may be clueless about your triggers. Therefore, it is best that you determine to help yourself with the help of our recommendations outlined below.

Headache Journal

To begin with, create a headache journal. The journal must have several columns, with diverse headings. These headings include, date of onset of migraine attack, exact time when it began and the exact time when it ended, intensity on a scale of one to ten, preceding symptoms, the triggers that set off the attack, various kinds of relief measures taken and the extent of relief (no relief, mild, moderate, or tremendous). After a couple of weeks or so, you should be able to witness a pattern. You will be able to comprehend your migraine disease better.

With regard to start and finish of the attack, ensure that you calculated the number of hours too. Your attacks may have lasted for the same duration each time, or varied.

The next column is about intensity. If you were able to complete your daily tasks without focusing too much on your pain, the attack could not be termed as severe. On the other hand, if the pain was so excruciating that it forced you to abandon everything and take rest, the attack could be deemed as extremely intense. Review your day before you rate your migraine attacks.

All right, what kind of symptoms preceded the actual onset? It is imperative that you take note of warning signs that precede every attack, for they will help you to take preventive or relief measures quickly.

Every migraine attack is different. Therefore, record all your information very carefully. For instance, you may have worsening migraines during weekends only. Then again, they may haunt the same side of your head all the time. Take note of the trigger factors. Something significant may have happened just before you began to experience this terrible pain in your head. It is not necessary that a sole trigger cause all your migraine attacks. There may be several triggers in your life. It is only now that you are beginning to associate them with your chronic malady. Regardless of the root cause being minor or major, take note of it. After all, you may be an extremely sensitive person, easily rattled by the mildest of circumstances. At least, the headache journal will help you work with this aspect of your personality too.

The last two columns focus on the kind of relief measures that you had taken after each migraine attack and the outcomes of those measures. For instance, your relief measures may include prescribed medications. Did you truly feel better after taking these pills? Did you experience any side effects? You need to provide answers to questions like these, for they will help your physician figure out what is exactly right for your condition. If you are taking other medications, which seem to clash with your migraine medications, mention them in your headache journal. Do not forget to mention other relief measures that you had taken after each attack, along with your prescribed drugs. For instance, you may have gone for a long walk, gone to bed in a darkened room, meditated, and so on. Every detail is important.

Finally, state the extent of relief that you obtained after the relief measures undertaken during each attack. It is possible that nothing helped during most of your attacks. Alternatively, you may have obtained significant relief through a single relief measure or a couple of actions. Whatever is the case, provide complete information about everything connected with your migraine disease. The journal is akin to a research project conducted on self, by self.

Food Triggers

As mentioned earlier, different foodstuffs can trigger a severe migraine attack. In fact, the list of foods to be avoided is quite lengthy. It is not necessary that every single foodstuff on the list is unsuitable for your constitution. You are well aware that every individual's constitution is different. However, some foodstuffs tend to cause all migraine sufferers to react in the same way. Try to figure out the common and specific foods that are not compatible with your brain and nervous system.

Once you manage to figure them out via your headache journal, you will be able to seek suitable substitutes for your food triggers. For instance, you may be extremely fond of tea and coffee. Now, there are all kinds of caffeinated, decaffeinated and herbal brands available. All that you will have to do is to switch over from caffeinated to decaffeinated and herbal varieties, since caffeine is bad for migraines. It is the same with fruits, vegetables, cheese, and so on. You need not worry that you will have to give up your favorites.

You might even ask your physician to suggest vitamin supplements as substitutes. For instance, if citrus fruits do not agree with you, vitamin C, along with other fruits and vegetables, would be a good alternative. You will comprehend that a particular foodstuff is a trigger, if you experience migraine within 24 hours of consuming it. Sometimes, the onset of the attack is even faster.

When you are purchasing groceries, please read the labels on bottles, tins and cans very carefully. You have to know what food additives are present in each recipe. To illustrate, sulfites are associated with French fries, jams, canned vegetables, precut vegetables, vegetable juice, wine, soft drinks, soup mixes, beer, shrimp, tea, dehydrated potatoes and dried fruit. Then again, MSG is found in chocolates. On some labels, it is displayed as yeast extract, soy protein, autolyzed yeast, natural flavoring, hydrolyzed vegetable, stock, broth, etc. Above all, when you go out to eat, ask for the relevant information from the waiter before you order anything from the menu.

Lifestyle

If you are constantly under stress, you need to figure out why. For instance, the thought of giving up certain foods may be upsetting you. However, you have no choice, since you are suffering from migraine disease. The good news is that you should be able to find substitutes for these foods.

It is also possible that you are prone to leading an unhealthy lifestyle. Then you will have to make some lifestyle changes. For instance, it would be good to chart out a routine for regular exercise or physical activities. Activities like brisk walking, swimming, taking up some kind of sport, etc., should work marvelously to reduce your stress levels. It is not necessary that you should go in for vigorous activities only. You may engage in mild-to-moderate exercise too. Oh, yes, ensure that you do not expose yourself to secondhand smoke too often, even if you do not smoke yourself.

Apart from food and exercise, you need to have adequate rest and sleep too. Do you get your required quota of seven to eight hours of sleep every night? If the answer is in the negative, you need to do something about your sleepless nights.

Medications

Do review your list of medications for various health concerns. It is quite possible that a newly added drug is causing migraine as a side effect.

Wrapping up!

A 'headache' is such a commonplace and acceptable occurrence in the modern, especially urban scenario, that you rarely give it a second thought when it actually hits you. All that you do is to swallow an analgesic with some water, or rest for a while, sincerely believing that you will feel normal again within a short while or so.

After all, you are aware of the cause too. It could relate to stress at work, financial issues at home, unexpected changes in routine, etc. However, if your head continues to throb for quite a while, along with enhanced sensitivity to sound and light, you should give serious thought to what is happening. It is possible that this is not the first time that you have experienced something like this. Instead of going in for self-diagnosis and self-medication, it would be best to consult a physician.

The exact causes of migraine disease remain confusing. Therefore, prevention may prove to be a problem. Yet, migraine sufferers may obtain tremendous relief through lifestyle changes, improved dietary regimens, prescribed medications and cultivation of a positive mindset.

At last, I would like to thank you for reading this book and hope that you will create a new healthier you!

www.ingramcontent.com/pod-product-compliance
Lightning Source LLC
Chambersburg PA
CBHW010918080626
46333CB00040B/579